CONTENTS

6 DAY express™
DIET PLAN

Accelerate your Slim in 6® results or get a quick weight loss tune-up with Beachbody's exclusive 6-Day Express weight loss plan.

We've all done it—put off losing weight before a wedding, vacation, or other special event until we're forced to do something drastic. That big day is quickly approaching, and suddenly you realize time is almost up for you to slim down.

That's why we created this program. We know this scenario happens all the time, so we wanted to provide some guidelines for shedding some fat and inches in one week, without jeopardizing your healthy lifestyle gains along the way.

That's right. In less than one week you can shed some serious weight by simply following this 6-Day Express Diet Plan. And best of all, this plan is totally natural—NO dangerous heart-pounding pills, magic potions, or fly-by-night fads. In some respects, this plan may resemble a fast, which can be a great way to cleanse the body, so long as you don't overdo it. Ever. That's why you need to limit the length of time you follow the program. It is extreme, for short-term extreme results.

Unfortunately, many people desperate for fast results make the mistake of doing anything it takes to lose weight. If "anything" to you means eating just three grapes while jogging from Cleveland to Miami, then weight is not the only thing you're going to lose. You'll sacrifice your health, hurt your metabolism, and probably just lose a lot of water. Now don't get us wrong; you will have to make sacrifices if you plan on shedding fat and inches in less than a week, but there is a better way to do it, both for short-term benefit and for avoiding long-term harm. The key is to follow a formula that is severe enough to get fast, optimal results, while at the same time allowing you to maintain your health and function at normal capacity. By following the 6-Day Express Diet Plan, this balance can be achieved!

© 2009 Beachbody. All rights reserved.

So What Is It Already?

The 6-Day Express Diet Plan consists of three very restrictive diet and exercise options to put your results on the fast track. Since each person has their own needs, limitations, and goals, we offer options of varying intensity. No matter which option you choose, it's important to note that this is an EXPRESS PLAN and not an EATING PLAN TO LIVE BY. Do not follow any of these plans longer than 6 days in any six-week cycle!

Warning: Seek the advice of your doctor before beginning any fast or diet program. Not advisable for pregnant or lactating women or anyone suffering from a medical condition.

HERE WE GO!

PLAN 1—GET IN THE ZONE

This is the most moderate of the three plans. Plan 1 is a balanced, healthy diet that is recommended for anyone new to dieting and exercise but still up for the challenge of the 6-Day Express.

PLAN 2—HIGH-PROTEIN EXPRESS

This plan adds protein and restricts carbohydrates to the bare minimum, similar to what bodybuilders do in order to prepare for competitions. Keep in mind that we don't recommend a diet this high in protein for long-term health. You are better off eating more complex carbs, your body's preferred fuel source. For 6 days, however, Plan 2 will force your body to use stored body fat for fuel while it ramps up your metabolism. A good short-term strategy!

PLAN 3—FIT-FOR-A-MINUTE...
AKA THE PHOTO SHOOT PLAN

The most extreme plan, which is similar to what bodybuilders and others needing to look their best go through when getting ready for a competition or photo shoot. This plan is very restrictive and difficult to follow. It also does not maximize your body's ability to perform. It is an extreme diet for when you absolutely, positively have to look your best for one special occasion.

Quick Tips for Best Results

WHEN TO EAT: 5–6 TIMES A DAY

Each plan spells it out for you, giving you six slots per day for eating. Essentially, you should get into the habit of eating every 3 hours or so while you're awake. In every plan of the 6-Day Express, you will usually wake up with a glass of water and then do some type of exercise before breakfast, so at times you may need to eat again in 2 hours. Given the size of many of the "meals," you probably won't have a problem with this. Finally, chewing food thoroughly will help "jump-start" digestion, making it easier on your gastrointestinal system.

SIZE MATTERS:

It's obvious that a person who weighs 300 pounds has different calorie and nutritional needs than a person who weighs 120 pounds, but weight is not the only factor. Differences in body composition (fat to muscle ratio) and metabolic rate means that there is no simple answer that works for everyone. Some people say a healthy body can survive at least 7 days with no food whatsoever. The point, however, isn't to "survive," but to tune up your body while maximizing its fat-burning mode in order to fast-track your results for 6 days with minimal consequence. You will be able to do the diet plan exactly as laid out, but you might benefit by altering it to suit your individual needs (i.e., body composition, size, activity level, etc.).

IS THIS ENOUGH FOOD FOR ME? HERE'S A WAY TO TELL:

1. Estimate your body-fat percentage. There are many ways to do this and most aren't perfectly accurate. Outside of having your body-fat percentage medically tested by your doctor or fitness professional, one of the most accurate measuring devices is also the cheapest: body-fat calipers (available at Beachbody.com or TeamBeachbody.com and many sporting goods stores). But any body-fat calculator can be used to give you an approximate figure to work from. These 6-day diets were designed for men with over 15% body fat and women with over 20% body fat. The reason is that you must have ample body fat stored to supply the balance of calories your body needs for energy while you are not feeding it as many calories as before. Keep in mind that "must" means just that. If you really feel like you need to eat more because your energy is too low, by all means do so.

© 2009 Beachbody. All rights reserved.

2. If you are a man with less than 15% body fat or a woman with less than 20% body fat, you will probably want to add calories in order to keep your workouts intense without your body feeding on its own muscle to support the demand for energy. Use the scale below to add the appropriate number of calories per day. The foods marked by an asterisk (*) in each plan are the ideal source for those additional calories.

Under 140 lbs.	add 100 cals per day
141–150 lbs.	add 200 cals per day
151–160 lbs.	add 300 cals per day
161–170 lbs.	add 400 cals per day
171–180 lbs.	add 500 cals per day
181–190 lbs.	add 600 cals per day
191–200 lbs.	add 700 cals per day
200+ lbs.	add 700 cals, plus another 100 cals for each 10 lbs. over 200 lbs.

WHEN TO WORK OUT:

We recommend that you do some cardio in the morning before you eat breakfast, and do your main, most intense workout later in the day. We do suggest specific workout times in each plan, but the bottom line is you should do your most challenging workout at whatever time of day you feel the strongest and most energetic. While there are advantages to working out at different times of the day, these advantages are superseded by your personal ability to push hard. When you are exercising just once a day, you should never compromise intensity just to get the workout done at a specific time. If you are exercising twice a day as we outline in the first two plans, we recommend that your toughest workout be later in the day when you've got more blood glycogen (sugar in the bloodstream) stored up. But again, the ultimate way to decide when to work out is based on when you can keep your intensity at its highest!

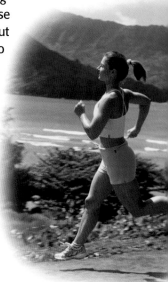

WHAT TYPES OF WORKOUTS TO FOLLOW:

While the 6-Day Express is designed around Slim in 6, it can be done with almost any exercise routine. (Note: Training for a marathon on this type of express diet would not work well—so try to make sure the intensity of the routine you pick does not push you outside of your capabilities at this time.)

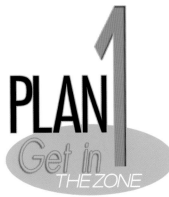

PLAN 1
Get in THE ZONE

This is the most moderate of the three plans. Plan 1 is a balanced, healthy diet recommended for anyone new to dieting and exercise but still up for the challenge of the 6-Day Express.

FOOD SUGGESTIONS ARE LISTED IN APPENDIX 2.

RECOMMENDATIONS ARE LISTED IN THE TABLE UNDER "FRUIT ONE," "FAT ONE," AND SO ON.

PLAN 1 SCHEDULE

WAKE-UP WATER

Have an 8–12 oz. glass of plain water to hydrate you when you wake up and before you begin your AM workout.

AM WORKOUT (CARDIO)

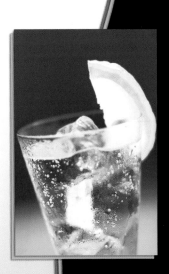

1. Do 20–60 minutes of easy to moderate intensity cardio before breakfast. If you are using Slim in 6, the cardio section of either the *Start It Up!* or *Ramp It Up!* routines is perfect. In your morning workout, you will want to skip the resistance work/exercise band section (which starts 20 minutes into *Ramp It Up!*, for instance).

2. Have breakfast within one hour of finishing your workout.

PRE-BREAKFAST WATER & SUPPLEMENTS

Have at least one 8 oz. glass of water with 2 Slimming Formula† tablets after you complete your AM workout, anytime prior to breakfast.

†As with any supplement, herb, or medication, do not use Slimming Formula while pregnant or lactating, or administer to a child without consulting a physician. Use this product only after consulting your physician about your specific health situation, especially if you are using any medications. Follow the directions as outlined for best results and do not exceed the recommended dosage.

© 2009 Beachbody. All rights reserved.

PLAN 1

Diet Plan 1:

Daily Calorie Count: Approximately 1,200 (115 grams carbohydrates, 92 grams protein, 40 grams fat)

BREAKFAST

Eat breakfast within one hour of finishing your AM workout. Approximately 325 calories (32 grams carbohydrates, 24 grams protein, 10 grams fat)

▲ **OPTION 1**

- Smoothie, with 1 scoop Beachbody's Whey Protein Powder,* one serving FRUIT ONE,* 1 tablespoon FAT ONE, in either 4 oz. of water or 4 oz. of soy or skim milk.* Mix in blender with a scoop of ice.

▲ **OPTION 2**

- 4 oz. MEAT (or MEAT SUBSTITUTE), grilled without oil*
- One serving FRUIT ONE*
- 1 tablespoon FAT ONE*
- 4 oz. soy or skim milk*

▲ **OPTION 3**

- 4 oz. MEAT (or MEAT SUBSTITUTE), grilled without oil*
- One serving GRAIN
- One serving FRUIT ONE
- One serving FAT ONE

PRE-SNACK WATER

Have at least one 8 oz. glass of water with (optional) lime or lemon added.

AM SNACK

Eat AM snack 1–2 hours after breakfast. Approximately 75 calories (18 grams carbohydrates)

- One serving FRUIT TWO

PRE-LUNCH WATER & SUPPLEMENTS

Have at least one 8 oz. glass of water with 2 Slimming Formula tablets and 1 ActiVit® capsule anytime before lunch.

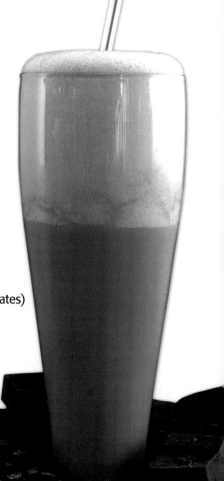

LUNCH

Eat lunch 1–2 hours after AM snack. Approximately 270 calories (14 grams carbohydrates, 23 grams protein, 16 grams fat)

- Salad
  - 1 cup SALAD with 1/4 cup SALAD INGREDIENT ONE* and 1 cup SALAD INGREDIENT TWO,* with 1 tablespoon balsamic vinaigrette (or equivalent dressing—no ranch, blue cheese, etc.)
  - 4 oz. of MEAT (or MEAT SUBSTITUTE), grilled without oil*

POST-LUNCH WATER

Have at least one 8 oz. glass of water anytime after lunch.

PM WORKOUT

Cardio plus strength training. High-intensity 30–60 minute workout, preferably with both cardio and resistance work (weight training) at higher intensity than morning workout.

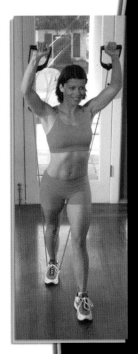

SLIM IN 6 OPTION:

Either *Ramp It Up!* or *Burn It Up!*

Note: Do the PM workout 2–3 hours after you've eaten, and if you have another meal left in the day, eat again within one hour of finishing the PM workout. If you do this workout before bed, then make sure you have a glass of water after finishing. Without enough water, you risk getting dehydrated while sleeping, which is when you are recovering and getting stronger. Your evening cup of tea before bed may help you get to sleep easily after working out.

PRE-SNACK WATER

Have at least one 8 oz. glass of water with (optional) lime or lemon added anytime before PM snack.

PM SNACK

Eat PM snack 1–3 hours after lunch. Approximately 230 calories (26 grams carbohydrates, 21 grams protein, 4 grams fat)

▲ OPTION 1
- Beachbody's Meal Replacement Shake (or equivalent) with 8 oz. soy or skim milk

▲ OPTION 2
- 130 calories of whole grain cereal (read nutrition panel as cereals vary) with 8 oz. soy or skim milk

© 2009 Beachbody. All rights reserved.

PLAN 1

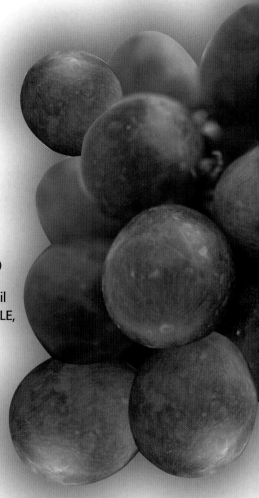

▲ **OPTION 3**

- 40/30/30 bar (up to 230 calories)

▲ **OPTION 4**

- 1/3 cup almonds, peanuts, or walnuts or pumpkin, sunflower, or sesame seeds raw

▲ **OPTION 5**

- 8 oz. vanilla or plain nonfat yogurt or soy yogurt

▲ **OPTION 6**

- 1/2 cup nonfat cottage cheese
- One serving FRUIT ONE or FRUIT TWO

▲ **OPTION 7**

- One serving GRAIN
- One serving FAT TWO

▲ **OPTION 8**

- 3 cups air-popped corn
- 1 cup soy or skim milk

PRE-DINNER WATER & SUPPLEMENTS

Have at least one 8 oz. glass of water with 2 Slimming Formula tablets and 1 ActiVit capsule anytime before dinner.

DINNER

Eat dinner 1–2 hours after your PM snack, or earlier, so you are done eating for the day within 3 hours of going to sleep! Approximately 280 calories (25 grams carbohydrates, 24 grams protein, 10 grams fat)

- 4 oz. MEAT (or MEAT SUBSTITUTE), grilled without oil
- 2 cups LEAFY GREEN VEGETABLE, steamed
- 2 oz. mustard
- One serving FRUIT ONE*

LATE SNACK

Approximately 0 calories

- 1 cup herbal tea

*Add quantities if necessary.

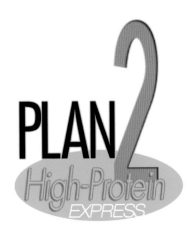

PLAN 2
High-Protein EXPRESS

In Plan 2, you consume mostly protein and restrict carbohydrates to a minimum, similar to what bodybuilders do in order to prepare for competitions. Keep in mind that we don't recommend a diet this high in protein for long-term health. In the short term, however, Plan 2 will force your body to use its stored body fat for fuel and also ramp up your metabolism.

FOOD SUGGESTIONS ARE LISTED IN APPENDIX 2.

RECOMMENDATIONS ARE LISTED IN THE TABLE UNDER "FRUIT ONE," "FAT ONE," AND SO ON.

PLAN 2 SCHEDULE

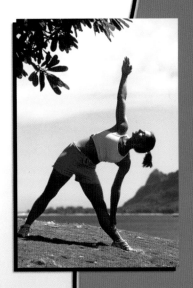

WAKE-UP WATER

Have an 8–12 oz. glass of plain water to hydrate you when you wake up and before you begin your AM workout.

AM WORKOUT (CARDIO)

1. Do 20–60 minutes of easy to moderate intensity cardio before breakfast. If you are using Slim in 6, the cardio section of either the *Start It Up!* or *Ramp It Up!* routines is perfect. In your morning workout, you will want to skip the resistance work/exercise band section (which starts 20 minutes into *Ramp It Up!*, for instance).

2. Have breakfast within one hour of finishing your workout.

PRE-BREAKFAST WATER & SUPPLEMENTS

Have at least one 8 oz. glass of water with 2 Slimming Formula tablets after you complete your AM workout, anytime prior to breakfast.

© 2009 Beachbody. All rights reserved.

PLAN 2

Diet Plan 2:

Daily Calorie Count: Approximately 1,200 (80 grams carbohydrates, 120 grams protein and 45 grams fat)

BREAKFAST

Eat breakfast within one hour of finishing your AM workout. Approximately 325 calories (32 grams carbohydrates, 24 grams protein, 10 grams fat)

▲ **OPTION 1**
- Smoothie, with 1 scoop Beachbody's Whey Protein Powder,* one serving FRUIT ONE,* 1 tablespoon FAT ONE, in either 4 oz. of water or 4 oz. of soy or skim milk.* Mix in blender with a scoop of ice.

▲ **OPTION 2**
- 4 oz. MEAT (or MEAT SUBSTITUTE), grilled without oil*
- One serving FRUIT ONE*
- 1 tablespoon FAT ONE*
- 4 oz. soy or skim milk*

PRE-SNACK WATER

Have at least one 8 oz. glass of water with (optional) lime or lemon added.

AM SNACK

Eat AM snack 1–2 hours after breakfast. Approximately 175 calories (12 grams carbohydrates, 22 grams protein, 3.5 grams fat)

▲ **OPTION 1**
- Small protein shake with 1 scoop Beachbody's Whey Protein Powder (or equivalent) in 4 oz. soy or skim milk*

▲ **OPTION 2**
- 4 oz. MEAT (or MEAT SUBSTITUTE), grilled without oil*
- 4 oz. soy or skim milk

PRE-LUNCH WATER & SUPPLEMENTS

Have at least one 8 oz. glass of water with 2 Slimming Formula tablets and 1 ActiVit capsule anytime before lunch.

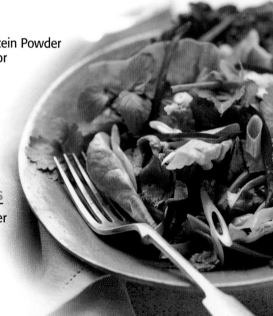

LUNCH

Eat lunch 1–2 hours after AM snack. Approximately 270 calories (14 grams carbohydrates, 23 grams protein, 16 grams fat)

- Salad
  - 1 cup SALAD with 1/4 cup SALAD INGREDIENT ONE* and 1 cup SALAD INGREDIENT TWO,* with 1 tablespoon balsamic vinaigrette (or equivalent dressing—no ranch, blue cheese, etc.)
- 4 oz. MEAT (or MEAT SUBSTITUTE), grilled without oil*

POST-LUNCH WATER

Have at least one 8 oz. glass of water anytime after lunch.

PM WORKOUT

Cardio plus strength training. Do a 30–60 minute workout, preferably with both cardio and resistance work (weight training), at high intensity.

SLIM IN 6 OPTION:
Either *Ramp It Up!* or *Burn It Up!*
Note: Do the PM workout 2–3 hours after you've eaten, and if you have another meal left in the day, eat again within one hour of finishing the PM workout. If you do this workout before bed, then make sure you have a glass of water after finishing. Without enough water, you risk getting dehydrated while sleeping, which is when you are recovering and getting stronger. Your evening cup of tea before bed may help you get to sleep easily after working out.

PRE-SNACK WATER

Have at least one 8 oz. glass of water with (optional) lime or lemon added anytime before PM snack.

PM SNACK

Eat PM snack 1–2 hours after lunch. Approximately 200 calories (6 grams carbohydrates, 26 grams protein, 6 grams fat)

- △ OPTION 1
  - Small protein shake with 1 heaping scoop Beachbody's Whey Protein Powder (or equivalent) in 5 oz. soy or skim milk*

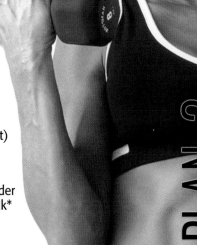

PLAN 2

© 2009 Beachbody. All rights reserved.

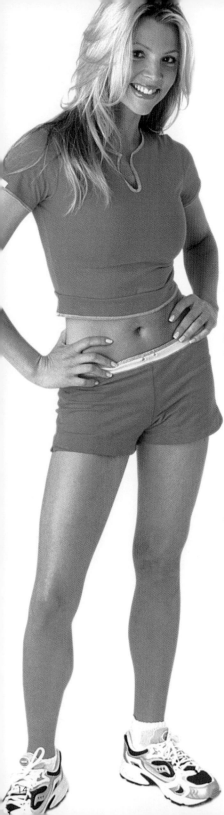

- 5 oz. MEAT (or MEAT SUBSTITUTE), grilled without oil*
- 5 oz. soy or skim milk

▲ OPTION 3

- 1/2 cup almonds, peanuts, or walnuts or pumpkin, sunflower, or sesame seeds, raw

PRE-DINNER WATER & SUPPLEMENTS

Have at least one 8 oz. glass of water with 2 Slimming Formula tablets and 1 ActiVit capsule anytime before dinner.

DINNER

Eat dinner 1–2 hours after your PM snack, or earlier, so you are done eating for the day within 3 hours of going to sleep! Approximately 230 calories (14 grams carbohydrates, 23 grams protein, 9 grams fat)

- 4 oz. MEAT (or MEAT SUBSTITUTE), grilled without oil*
- 2 cups LEAFY GREEN VEGETABLE, steamed*
- 2 oz. mustard

LATE SNACK

Approximately 0 calories

- 1 cup herbal tea

*Add quantities if necessary.

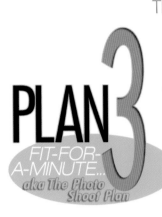

PLAN 3

FIT-FOR-A-MINUTE...
aka The Photo Shoot Plan

This is the most extreme plan, similar to what bodybuilders and others wanting to look their best on a specific day will go through when getting ready for a competition or photo shoot. This plan is very restrictive and difficult to follow. It does not maximize your body's ability to perform. It is an extreme diet for when you absolutely, positively have to look "shredded." But please understand, it's not healthy. It's not good for you. It's not something to do often.

Warning: Do not attempt this plan unless you are in very good health. Under no circumstances should you undertake this if you have high blood pressure or a heart ailment of any kind!

The plan is two-tiered. First you start with a 3-day cleanse in order to rid your body of unwanted, undigested food and toxins. Next are 3 days designed to "wring out your body" by eating only lean protein, very little fat, carbs, and even very little water. Like we said—it's not healthy, but if you need that one shredded, ripped day, this is what the pros do.

FOOD SUGGESTIONS ARE LISTED IN APPENDIX 2.

RECOMMENDATIONS ARE LISTED IN THE TABLE UNDER "FRUIT ONE," "FAT ONE," AND SO ON.

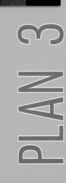

PLAN 3

© 2009 Beachbody. All rights reserved.

A slightly modified veggie fast, where you'll mainly be eating raw foods—plants and grains—in order to cleanse your system. Extra water is fine for these three days. Exercise may be a struggle, so back off if you need to.

WAKE-UP WATER

Have one 8–12 oz. glass of plain water to hydrate you when you wake up and before you begin your AM workout.

AM WORKOUT (OPTIONAL IN PLAN 3)

1. If you want to exercise, do 20–30 minutes of low-intensity yoga, cardio, or stretching. Make sure to warm up thoroughly before doing any difficult movements.
2. Have breakfast within one hour of finishing your workout.

PRE-BREAKFAST WATER

Have at least one 8 oz. glass of water after you complete your AM workout, anytime prior to breakfast.

Diet Plan 3, Part One:

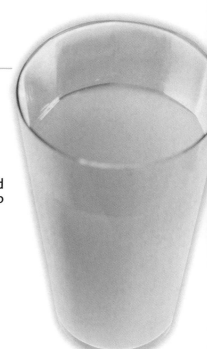

BREAKFAST

Eat breakfast within one hour of waking up or exercising.

▲ OPTION 1
- Protein shake with 1 scoop Beachbody's Whey Protein Powder in 4 oz. water*

▲ OPTION 2
- 1/2 cup fruit juice (no sugar added and freshly squeezed if possible) or 1/2 cup vegetable juice (fresh if possible—low sodium if purchased)

PRE-SNACK WATER

Have at least one 8 oz. glass of water with (optional) lime or lemon added.

AM SNACK

Eat AM snack 1–2 hours after breakfast.

▲ OPTION 1
- 1 scoop Beachbody's Meal Replacement Shake in 8 oz. water*

▲ OPTION 2
- 1/2 cup fruit juice (no sugar added and freshly squeezed if possible) or

1/2 cup vegetable juice (fresh if possible—low sodium if purchased)

Have at least one 8 oz. glass of water and 1 ActiVit capsule anytime before lunch.

LUNCH

Eat lunch 1–2 hours after AM snack.

- Salad
  - 1 cup SALAD,* 1 cup SALAD INGREDIENT ONE,* and 1 cup SALAD INGREDIENT TWO* with spices and balsamic vinegar
  - 1 tablespoon raw seeds or nuts
- 1 cup wild rice (cooked, no additives) or 1 cup cooked oatmeal*

POST-LUNCH WATER

Have at least one 8 oz. glass of water anytime after lunch.

PM WORKOUT

At moderate intensity, do a 20–60 minute workout that has both cardio and resistance work. Start 2–3 hours after your most recent meal and eat again within one hour of finishing.

SLIM IN 6 OPTION:
Start It Up!, Ramp It Up!, or *Keep It Up!*

PRE-SNACK WATER

Have at least one 8 oz. glass of water with (optional) lime or lemon added anytime before PM snack.

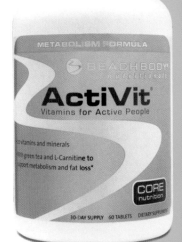

PM SNACK

- 1 cup SALAD INGREDIENT ONE or SALAD INGREDIENT TWO, raw*
- 1 tablespoon raw seeds or nuts
- 1/2 cup fruit juice (no sugar added and freshly squeezed if possible) or 1/2 cup vegetable juice (fresh if possible—low sodium if purchased)

PRE-DINNER WATER & SUPPLEMENTS

Have at least one 8 oz. glass of water and 1 ActiVit capsule anytime before dinner.

PLAN 3

© 2009 Beachbody. All rights reserved.

DINNER

Eat dinner 1–2 hours after your PM snack, or earlier, so you are done eating for the day within 3 hours of going to sleep!

- 2 cups LEAFY GREEN VEGETABLE, steamed*
- 1/2 cup wild/brown rice or oatmeal, cooked

LATE PM SNACK

- 1 cup herbal tea
- One 8 oz. glass of water
- Suck on ice
- Breathe in steam for 10 minutes
- Suck on a sponge (if you don't think this is a joke, you'd better make it a very clean sponge!)

Part Two—GET RIPPED!

High protein and low everything else, INCLUDING WATER, will shed unsightly fat and wring the water out of your system in order to show more definition. Definitely should not be pushed outside of 3 days, as your body cannot live long on this diet. We doubt you'll want to. After 3 days, that damp sponge will no doubt seem appealing. On this diet, YOU MAY NOT EAT OR DRINK ANYTHING ELSE, INCLUDING WATER, except 2 cups per day of coffee or tea (as they are diuretics—but no additives). However, based on your size, you may vary the portion size.

You must purchase a POTASSIUM supplement, which can be found at any market and should only cost a few dollars. Potassium supplementation will ensure that your electrolyte balance doesn't get too far out of whack and will also help you shed excess sodium from your system that can make you look bloated. Do not add any salt to your food during this time.

During your last 24 hours, do not drink any water. If you are parched, just have enough to moisten you mouth. Sucking on ice (seriously) can help you if you're feeling very thirsty.

Also, try and keep your veggie intake to those with lower water contents.

HERE IS A LIST OF RECOMMENDED VEGGIES:		AND HERE ARE A FEW TO AVOID (UNLESS YOU WANT TO CHEAT):	
GREEN BEANS	BRUSSELS SPROUTS	SQUASH	SPINACH
BROCCOLI	CAULIFLOWER	TOMATOES	ZUCCHINI
PEAS		BOK CHOY	LETTUCE (ALL TYPES)

Feel like this is crazy? Here are some inspiring words from someone who's gone through it many times, bodybuilder Patricia Beyeler:

"By now, you can't add muscle if you are not already there, but you can make sure your sodium level is extremely low and your potassium is higher at this time. Only potassium pills can help (no bananas). Eat protein only in the form of lean meat, egg whites, and protein shakes with water only, no protein bars. Tanning is great the night before (I do this even with my nice brown skin—LOL!). Tanning sucks out the excess water somewhat like a diuretic would. Eat only a palm-sized portion of brown rice prior to the shoot, and only if you are going to show various routines or exercises so you need more energy. No water over the last 24 hours, just enough to wet your whistle. Sorry, but this is extreme."

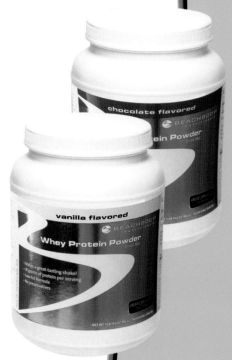

WAKE-UP WATER

Have a glass of water when you wake up. Remember, though, none on the last day, but you can rinse out your mouth after brushing your teeth.

AM WORKOUT (OPTIONAL IN PLAN 3)

You can't add much at this stage of the game. If you want to do something to feel good, make it low intensity.

Diet Plan 3, Part Two:

BREAKFAST

Eat breakfast within one hour of waking up or exercising.

△ **OPTION 1**
- Protein shake with 1 scoop Beachbody's Whey Protein Powder, in 4 oz. water* with 200 mg. of potassium

△ **OPTION 2**
- 6 egg whites with herbs (absolutely no salt added)*

AM SNACK

Eat AM snack 1–2 hours after breakfast.

△ **OPTION 1**
- Protein shake with 1 scoop Beachbody's Whey Protein Powder, in 4 oz. water*

△ **OPTION 2**
- 6 egg whites with herbs (absolutely no salt added)*

PLAN 3

© 2009 Beachbody. All rights reserved.

Have at least one 8 oz. glass of water anytime before lunch with 200 mg. potassium. On the last day, drink only enough to get the pills down.

LUNCH

Eat lunch 1–2 hours after AM snack.

- 4–8 oz. MEAT (or MEAT SUBSTITUTE), grilled without oil
- 1 cup LEAFY GREEN VEGETABLE
- WORKOUT OPTION. If you are doing a hard afternoon workout, add 1 cup wild rice (cooked, no additives) or 1 cup cooked oatmeal*

PM WORKOUT

At moderate intensity, 20–60 minute workout that has both cardio and resistance work. Start 2–3 hours after your most recent meal and eat again within one hour of finishing.

SLIM IN 6 OPTION:
Start It Up!, Ramp It Up!, or Keep It Up!

PRE-SNACK WATER & SUPPLEMENTS

Have at least one 8 oz. glass of water anytime after lunch with 200 mg. potassium. On the last day, drink only enough to get the pills down.

PM SNACK

Skip during last 24 hours.

- 4 oz. MEAT (or MEAT SUBSTITUTE), grilled without oil
- 1 cup LEAFY GREEN VEGETABLE

PRE-DINNER WATER & SUPPLEMENTS

Have at least one 8 oz. glass of water anytime after lunch with 200 mg. potassium. On the last day, drink only enough to get the pills down.

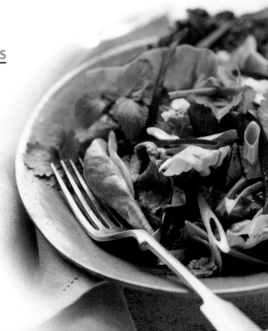

DINNER

Eat dinner 1–2 hours after your PM snack, or earlier, so you are done eating for the day within 3 hours of going to sleep!

- 4–8 oz. MEAT (or MEAT SUBSTITUTE), grilled without oil
- 1 cup LEAFY GREEN VEGETABLE

LATE PM SNACK

- Suck on ice (and you thought we were kidding, huh?)

*Add quantities if necessary.

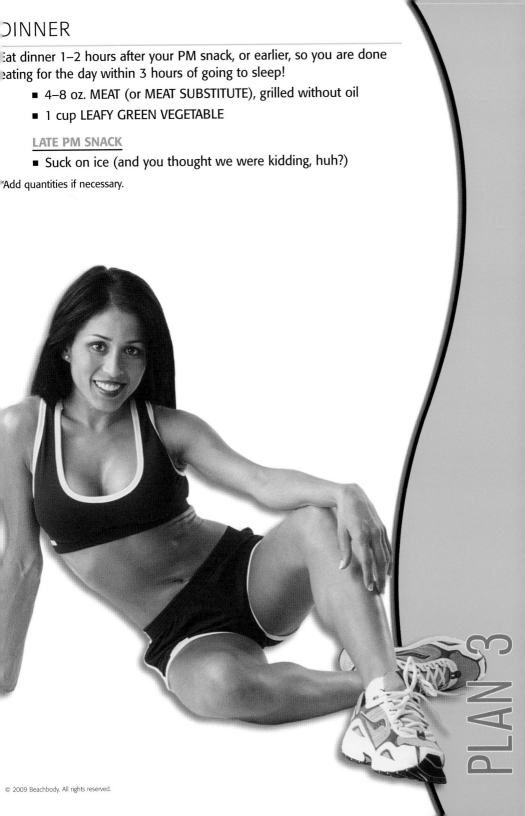

PLAN 3

© 2009 Beachbody. All rights reserved.

6-DAY EXPRESS NOTES

ALCOHOL—Stock up, 'cause you're gonna need it—wait a sec—you can't have any at all.

COFFEE AND TEA—These beverages have no calories unless you add things to them. So you can drink them, but only without the added calories. Keep in mind that both promote some amount of dehydration, so extra water should be consumed throughout the day if you drink coffee or tea (except during the Get Ripped phase of Plan 3). Also, on Plan 3 you'll find that caffeine has a heightened effect due to the types of foods you are eating (or lack thereof). You should consider cutting your caffeine way down, if not out, while doing Plan 3, or at least switching to green tea.

FLAX AND HEMPSEED—Each plan is going to require a trip to the market. Two items you may not be used to are flax and hempseed. Flaxseed provides your body with essential fatty acids, and raw seeds (as opposed to flaxseed oil) are a great source of fiber as well. You can eat the seeds whole, but most people prefer to grind them up and add them to a shake. Either way is fine. You can grind your flaxseeds in a standard coffee grinder or sprinkle them on your salad. Certain stores now sell ground flaxseed as well. Using flax, fish, or any omega-3 oil is an appropriate (and easier) substitute, whether in capsule or liquid form. Keep in mind that you'll be missing out on some fiber. You can replace this with a spoonful of psyllium husk if you choose.

FRUIT JUICE—Should be 1/2 cup fruit juice (no sugar added and freshly squeezed if possible) diluted with 1/2 cup of water.

GRAINS—Grains can be soothing on the digestive system and are sometimes used during fasts.

POTASSIUM—In supplement form, potassium is only needed for the last 3 days of Plan 3. Potassium, a mineral, assists in muscle contraction and in maintaining fluid and electrolyte balance in body cells. Potassium is important in sending nerve impulses as well as releasing energy from protein, fat, and carbohydrates during metabolism. During the Get Ripped phase of Plan 3, you have an increased need for potassium because you are forcing your body to excrete excess water. Potassium is necessary for water balance and is found inside every cell in your body. The potassium inside the cells balances the sodium outside the cells to maintain pressure and water balance in the body. A higher sodium intake increases fluid retention outside your cells. Increasing your potassium intake will cause that extra sodium to be excreted.

PROTEIN POWDER AND MEAL REPLACEMENT SHAKES—We also recommend Beachbody's Whey Protein Powder and Meal Replacement Shake, but you don't have to use our products. There are many products on the market, so feel free to substitute whatever is convenient. We just happen to know the content and quality of our products, which is why we recommend them with the 6-Day Express Diet Plan.

SOFT DRINKS—C'mon, whaddaya, a comedian? Nice try. Even diet soft drinks are off, as they contain zero food value and are loaded with controversial ingredients.

6-DAY EXPRESS NOTES

SPORTS DRINKS AND JUICES—These are not allowed and will interfere with your results. They certainly have a place in a sound long-term nutrition and fitness program, but are superfluous calories during the 6-Day Express Diet Plan and should be avoided.

VEGETABLE JUICE— One cup of fresh juice, if possible (low sodium if purchased).

WATER—There are water guidelines in the plans, but you are able to add water as necessary (except during the Get Ripped phase of Plan 3). Some carbonated water is okay, but make most of your water flat, as a steady diet of carbonated water will upset your body's phosphorus levels. Do not drink less water than what is advised.

CAN I DO IT LONGER THAN 6 DAYS?—We do not recommend using the 6-Day Express Diet Plan longer than 6 days. For one, it could be dangerous, and two, you run the risk of slowing your metabolism from under-eating, which could reverse your results. You can, however, keep eating in this fashion by adding more calories from similar types of foods.

CAN I DO THE 2-DAY FAST?—Beachbody's 2-Day Fast Start Plan is suggested to kick off Plans 1 and 2, but not Plan 3, since Plan 3 is a cleansing diet and similar to a fast anyway. For cleansing purposes, it is possible to add the 2-Day Fast Start Plan to the end of Plans 1 and 2 as well. We highly recommend that you stop (or at least reduce) exercising if you fast, and schedule this fast over two days when you don't have much to do, since you won't have much energy. For more information on the 2-Day Fast Start Plan and Beachbody's 2-Day Fast Formula, go to Beachbody.com or TeamBeachbody.com.

Keep in mind this 6-Day Express Diet Plan was designed to allow for maximum weight loss in a short period of time. Deviating from any of the suggestions provided will more than likely have a negative effect on your results.

We never said it was going to be a cakewalk (sorry, probably wrong choice of words). But we do say that you will rapidly accelerate the weight loss process if you stick to one of these 6-day plans. Chances are, you're here because you need to lose weight fast, and you want to do it in the healthiest possible way. With that in mind, take comfort in knowing that our fitness and diet experts have spent countless hours creating safe and effective plans that WILL PROVIDE THE FAST RESULTS YOU NEED.

Of course, results will vary. You will continue to lose or gain weight after completing the 6-Day Express Diet depending on your exercise and eating habits. Remember, you can continue to maintain your new physique with Debbie Siebers' *Keep It Up!* workout, the perfect way to stay motivated and sustain your level of fitness and health.

© 2009 Beachbody. All rights reserved.

FOOD LIST

FRUIT ONE

Banana, 1/2   Strawberries, sliced, 1 cup
Raspberries, 1 cup   Blackberries, 3/4 cup
Blueberries, 3/4 cup   Boysenberries, 1 cup

FRUIT TWO

Apple, 1 medium   Orange, 1 medium
Pear, 1 medium   Kiwi, 1 medium
Nectarine, 1 medium   Peach, 1 medium
Grapes, 1 cup   Pineapple, 1 cup
Melon, 1 cup   Grapefruit, 1/2 large
Tangerines, 2 small   Mango, 1/2 small
Papaya, 1/2 small   Plums, 2 small

SALAD

Spinach   Lettuce (any except iceberg)
Endive

SALAD INGREDIENT ONE

Chopped green onions   Cucumber
Celery   Parsley
Arugula

SALAD INGREDIENT TWO

Bell pepper   Mushrooms
Broccoli   Cauliflower
Green string beans   Carrot
Radish   Asparagus

LEAFY GREEN VEGETABLE

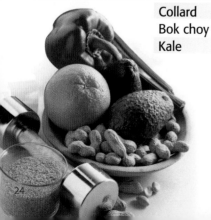

Collard   Cabbage
Bok choy   Brussels sprouts
Kale   Chard

FOOD LIST

GRAIN

Cereal (less than 7 grams of sugar per serving), 3/4 cup
Cooked oatmeal, 1/2 cup
Whole grain bread (no enriched flour), 1 slice
Flourless bread, 1 slice

MEAT

Chicken breast (skinless)	Lean steak
Fish	Lean lamb
Turkey	Pork tenderloin

MEAT SUBSTITUTE

Tofu	Tempeh
Seitan	Cottage cheese (nonfat), 1/2 cup
Soy cheese, 3 slices	Egg whites, 6
Egg substitute (plain), 3/4 cup	Hummus, 1/4 cup
Plain yogurt (nonfat), 1 cup	Soy yogurt, 1 cup

Beans, Lentils, or Soybeans (cooked), 3/4 cup
Soy burger (less than 5 grams of fat per serving)

FAT ONE

Ground flaxseed (recommended), 1 tablespoon
Flaxseed oil (capsule okay), 1 tablespoon
Fish oil (capsule okay)
Any omega-3 supplement
Olive or Canola oil, 1 tablespoon
Safflower, Borage, Flax, Evening Primrose, Sunflower,
or Hemp oil, 1 tablespoon

FAT TWO

Olives, 16
Avocado, 1/4
Peanut or Almond butter, 1 tablespoon
Almonds, Peanuts, or Walnuts, 2 tablespoons (1/8 cup, raw)
Sunflower, Sesame, or Pumpkin seeds, 2 tablespoons (1/8 cup, raw)

© 2009 Beachbody. All rights reserved.

JOURNAL DAY 1

Goals/Resolutions for the next 6 days:

DIET PLAN NUMBER:
Wake-Up Water:
AM Workout (Cardio):
Pre-Breakfast Water & Supplements:
Breakfast:

Pre-Snack Water:
AM Snack:
Pre-Lunch Water & Supplements:
Lunch:

Post-Lunch Water:
PM Workout (Cardio plus Strength Training):
Pre-Snack Water:
PM Snack:
Pre-Dinner Water & Supplements:
Dinner:

Late Snack:
Comments:

JOURNAL DAY 2

Goals/Resolutions for the day:

Wake-Up Water:
AM Workout (Cardio):
Pre-Breakfast Water & Supplements:
Breakfast:

Pre-Snack Water:
AM Snack:
Pre-Lunch Water & Supplements:
Lunch:

Post-Lunch Water:
PM Workout (Cardio plus Strength Training):
Pre-Snack Water:
PM Snack:
Pre-Dinner Water & Supplements:
Dinner:

Late Snack:
Comments:

© 2009 Beachbody. All rights reserved.

JOURNAL DAY 3

Goals/Resolutions for the day:

Wake-Up Water:
AM Workout (Cardio):
Pre-Breakfast Water & Supplements:
Breakfast:

Pre-Snack Water:
AM Snack:
Pre-Lunch Water & Supplements:
Lunch:

Post-Lunch Water:
PM Workout (Cardio plus Strength Training):
Pre-Snack Water:
PM Snack:
Pre-Dinner Water & Supplements:
Dinner:

Late Snack:
Comments:

JOURNAL DAY 4

Goals/Resolutions for the day:

Wake-Up Water:

AM Workout (Cardio):

Pre-Breakfast Water & Supplements:

Breakfast:

Pre-Snack Water:

AM Snack:

Pre-Lunch Water & Supplements:

Lunch:

Post-Lunch Water:

PM Workout (Cardio plus Strength Training):

Pre-Snack Water:

PM Snack:

Pre-Dinner Water & Supplements:

Dinner:

Late Snack:

Comments:

© 2009 Beachbody. All rights reserved.

Goals/Resolutions for the day:

Wake-Up Water:
AM Workout (Cardio):
Pre-Breakfast Water & Supplements:
Breakfast:

Pre-Snack Water:
AM Snack:
Pre-Lunch Water & Supplements:
Lunch:

Post-Lunch Water:
PM Workout (Cardio plus Strength Training):
Pre-Snack Water:
PM Snack:
Pre-Dinner Water & Supplements:
Dinner:

Late Snack:
Comments:

JOURNAL DAY 6

Goals/Resolutions for the day:

Wake-Up Water:
AM Workout (Cardio):
Pre-Breakfast Water & Supplements:
Breakfast:

Pre-Snack Water:
AM Snack:
Pre-Lunch Water & Supplements:
Lunch:

Post-Lunch Water:
PM Workout (Cardio plus Strength Training):
Pre-Snack Water:
PM Snack:
Pre-Dinner Water & Supplements:
Dinner:

Late Snack:
Comments:

© 2009 Beachbody. All rights reserved.

BEFORE AND AFTER STATS

BEFORE	AFTER

DATE: _____

WEIGHT: _____

CHEST: _____ "

WAIST: _____ "

HIPS: _____ "

**RIGHT
MID-THIGH:** _____ "

**LEFT
MID-THIGH:** _____ "

**RIGHT
UPPER ARM:** _____ "
(FLEXED, MEASURED AT THE PEAK OF THE BICEP)

**LEFT
UPPER ARM:** _____ "
(FLEXED, MEASURED AT THE PEAK OF THE BICEP)

DATE: _____

WEIGHT: _____

CHEST: _____ "

WAIST: _____ "

HIPS: _____ "

**RIGHT
MID-THIGH:** _____ "

**LEFT
LEFT MID-THIGH:** _____ "

**RIGHT
UPPER ARM:** _____ "
(FLEXED, MEASURED AT THE PEAK OF THE BICEP)

**LEFT
UPPER ARM:** _____ "
(FLEXED, MEASURED AT THE PEAK OF THE BICEP)